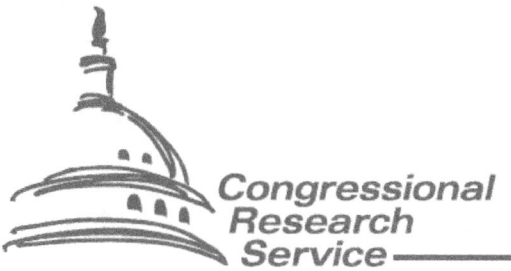

Congressional
Research
Service

Prescription Drug Monitoring Programs

Kristin M. Finklea
Specialist in Domestic Security

Erin Bagalman
Analyst in Health Policy

Lisa N. Sacco
Analyst in Illicit Drugs and Crime Policy

July 10, 2012

Congressional Research Service
7-5700
www.crs.gov
R42593

CRS Report for Congress
Prepared for Members and Committees of Congress

Summary

In the midst of national concern over illicit drug use and abuse, prescription drug abuse has been identified as the United States' fastest growing drug problem. Nearly all prescription drugs involved in overdoses are originally prescribed by a physician (rather than, for example, being stolen from pharmacies). Thus, attention has been directed toward preventing the diversion of prescription drugs after the prescriptions are dispensed.

Prescription drug monitoring programs (PDMPs) maintain statewide electronic databases of prescriptions dispensed for controlled substances (i.e., prescription drugs of abuse that are subject to stricter government regulation). Information collected by PDMPs may be used to support access to and legitimate medical use of controlled substances; identify or prevent drug abuse and diversion; facilitate the identification of prescription drug-addicted individuals and enable intervention and treatment; outline drug use and abuse trends to inform public health initiatives; or educate individuals about prescription drug use, abuse, and diversion as well as about PDMPs.

How PDMPs are organized and operated varies among states. Each state determines which agency houses the PDMP; which controlled substances must be reported; which types of dispensers are required to submit data (e.g., pharmacies); how often data are collected; who may access information in the PDMP database (e.g., prescribers, dispensers, or law enforcement); the circumstances under which the information may (or must) be accessed; and what enforcement mechanisms are in place for noncompliance.

PDMP costs may vary widely, with startup costs ranging from $450,000 to over $1.5 million and annual operating costs ranging from $125,000 to nearly $1.0 million. States finance PDMPs using monies from a variety of sources including the state general fund, prescriber and pharmacy licensing fees, state controlled substance registration fees, health insurers' fees, direct-support organizations, state grants, and/or federal grants. The federal government has established two grant programs aimed at supporting state PDMPs: The Harold Rogers PDMP grant, administered by the Department of Justice, and the National All Schedules Prescription Electronic Reporting Act of 2005 (NASPER) grant, administered by the Department of Health and Human Services. The Harold Rogers PDMP received $7.0 million in appropriations for FY2012; NASPER last received appropriations (of $2.0 million) in FY2010.

State PDMPs vary widely with respect to whether or how information contained in the database is shared with other states. While some states do not have measures in place allowing interstate sharing of information, others have specific practices for sharing. An effort is ongoing to facilitate information sharing using prescription monitoring information exchange (PMIX) architecture. Currently, there are no national level standards for state PDMP information sharing and interoperability. Legislation has been introduced in the 112th Congress that would take up these issues (see, for example, Section 1141 of the Food and Drug Administration Safety and Innovation Act (S. 3187), the Medicare and Medicaid FAST Act (H.R. 3399, S. 1251), and ID MEDS Act (H.R. 4292, S. 2254)).

The available evidence suggests that PDMPs are effective in reducing the time required for drug diversion investigations, changing prescribing behavior, reducing "doctor shopping," and reducing prescription drug abuse; however, research on the effectiveness of PDMPs is limited. Assessments of effectiveness may also take into consideration potential unintended consequences of PDMPs, such as limiting access to medications for legitimate use or pushing drug diversion activities over the border into a neighboring state. Experts suggest that PDMP effectiveness might be improved by increasing the timeliness, completeness, consistency, and accessibility of the data.

Current policy issues that might come before Congress include the role of state PDMPs in the federal prescription drug abuse strategy and the role of the federal government in interstate data-sharing and interoperability. While establishment and enhancement of PDMPs enjoy broad support, stakeholders express concerns about health care versus law enforcement uses of PDMP data (particularly with regard to protection of personally identifiable health information) and maintaining access to medication for patients with legitimate medical needs.

Contents

Tables

Contacts

Introduction

In the midst of national concern over illicit drug use and abuse, prescription drug abuse has been identified as the United States' fastest growing drug problem.[1] Seven million individuals aged 12 or older (2.7% of this population) were current nonmedical[2] users of prescription—or psychotherapeutic—drugs in 2010.[3] Over 1 million emergency department visits involved nonmedical use of pharmaceuticals in 2009.[4]

Leading the spike in prescription drug abuse is an "epidemic of prescription painkiller abuse. Nearly three out of four prescription drug overdoses are caused by prescription painkillers" or opiods.[5] Prescription drug overdoses caused 20,044 deaths in the United States in 2008; of these, 74% (14,800) involved opioid pain relievers.[6] Of those individuals who used prescription painkillers non-medically in 2010, nearly three-quarters received the drugs from a friend or relative—either for free, through a purchase, or via stealing the drugs.[7] Aside from prescription painkillers such as oxycodone, other commonly abused medications include benzodiazepines and amphetamine-like drugs.

Florida has been cited as an epicenter of prescription drug abuse. Florida doctors prescribe "10 times more oxycodone pills than every other state in the country combined."[8] Data indicate that 2,488 individuals in Florida died from prescription drugs in 2009[9]—averaging 6.8 prescription drug-related deaths per day. Many have cited the burgeoning number of legal pain management

---

[1] Office of National Drug Control Policy, *Prescription Drug Abuse*, http://www.whitehouse.gov/ondcp/prescription-drug-abuse. Prescription drugs of abuse are often divided into the categories of *pain relievers* (e.g., oxycodone), central nervous system *stimulants* (e.g., amphetamine), and central nervous system *depressants* (e.g., benzodiazepines). Pain relievers that are subject to abuse may be called *narcotics* or *opioids*. Central nervous system depressants may be further divided into *tranquilizers* (also called *anxiolytics*, used to reduce anxiety) and *sedatives* (also called *sedative-hypnotics*, used to induce sleep). The term *psychotherapeutics* is sometimes used to capture all of these categories.

[2] *Nonmedical use* of prescription drugs occurs when the drugs are used without a prescription or solely for the feeling they cause. Terms such as *misuse, abuse, dependence,* and *addiction* are often used interchangeably with nonmedical use, although each term may have its own definition within a specific context.

[3] U.S. Department of Health and Human Services, Substance Abuse and Mental Health Services Administration, *Results from the 2010 National Survey on Drug Use and Health Summary of National Findings*, September 2011, http://www.oas.samhsa.gov/NSDUH/2k10NSDUH/2k10Results.htm#Ch2. Hereafter: *2010 National Survey on Drug Use and Health*. According to the survey, "current" was defined as using the drug within the past month.

[4] U.S. Department of Health and Human Services, Substance Abuse and Mental Health Services Administration, *Drug Abuse Warning Network, 2009 National Estimates of Drug-Related Emergency Department Visits*, August 2011, http://www.samhsa.gov/data/2k11/DAWN/2k9DAWNED/HTML/DAWN2k9ED.htm#High6. These are the most recent data from the Drug Abuse Warning Network.

[5] Centers for Disease Control and Prevention, *Policy Impact Prescription Painkiller Overdoses*, December 19, p. 2011, http://www.cdc.gov/homeandrecreationalsafety/rxbrief/. Hereafter: *Policy Impact Prescription Painkiller Overdoses.*

[6] Centers for Disease Control and Prevention, *Vital Signs Overdoses of Prescription Opioid Pain Relievers - United States, 1999-2008*, November 4, 2011, http://www.cdc.gov/mmwr/preview/mmwrhtml/mm6043a4.htm. These are the most recent data available.

[7] 2010 National Survey on Drug Use and Health.

[8] Greg Allen, "The 'Oxy Express': Florida's Drug Abuse Epidemic," *NPR*, March 2, 2011, http://www.npr.org/2011/03/02/134143813/the-oxy-express-floridas-drug-abuse-epidemic.

[9] Florida Department of Law Enforcement, *Drugs Identified in Deceased Persons by Florida Medical Examiners*, 2009 Report, June 2010, http://www.fdle.state.fl.us/Content/getdoc/742e2162-c1de-4ecd-bce4-857a32c6f42e/2009-Drug-Report.aspx.

clinics and illegitimate clinics (or "pill mills") as contributing to the epidemic.[10] While Florida has been noted for its legitimate and illegitimate prescription drug distribution, states throughout the nation face the same threats from prescription drug abuse and have taken measures to prevent and treat the abuse as well as to ensure the operation of legitimate prescription drug dispensaries and pharmacies.

Nearly all prescription drugs involved in overdoses are originally prescribed by a physician (rather than, for example, being stolen from pharmacies).[11] Thus, attention has been directed toward preventing the diversion of prescription drugs after the prescriptions are dispensed. Prescription drug monitoring programs (PDMPs) maintain statewide electronic databases of dispensed prescriptions for controlled substances. PDMP information can aid those in law enforcement and/or health care in identifying patterns of prescribing, dispensing, or receiving controlled substances that may indicate abuse.[12]

For over a decade, Congress has provided financial support for state-level PDMPs using electronic databases. In 2002, Congress established the Harold Rogers PDMP grant, administered by the Department of Justice (DOJ), to help law enforcement, regulatory entities, and public health officials analyze data on prescriptions for controlled substances. Three years later, Congress passed the National All Schedules Prescription Electronic Reporting Act of 2005 (NASPER) requiring the Secretary of Health and Human Services (HHS) to award grants to states to establish or improve PDMPs.

The 112th Congress has demonstrated a particular interest in facilitating interoperability among state-level PDMPs, as well as in establishing national programs.[13] While the majority of PDMP-related proposals in the 112th Congress would focus on enhancing state-level databases and interstate information sharing, others have suggested establishing a national system. A related issue that policymakers may consider is whether PDMPs and their interstate information sharing platforms adequately protect personally identifiable and related health information and whether they can ensure that patients with legitimate medical needs have access to prescriptions. Congress may also exercise oversight with respect to the role of PDMPs in the Administration's action plan to combat the prescription drug epidemic;[14] policymakers may question the extent to which the Office of National Drug Control Policy (ONDCP), along with the other relevant departments and agencies, has taken steps to accomplish these PDMP-related goals laid out in the plan.

This report provides an overview of PDMPs, including their operation, enforcement mechanisms, costs, and financing. It also examines the effectiveness of PDMPs and outlines federal grants supporting PDMPs. Finally, this report discusses relevant considerations for policymakers, such as interstate data sharing, interoperability, and protection of health information.

---

[10] Legislation has been introduced in the 112th Congress (e.g., the Pill Mill Crackdown Act of 2011 (H.R. 1065, S. 1760)) that would, among other things, provide specific penalties for operating a pill mill.

[11] *Policy Impact Prescription Painkiller Overdoses.*

[12] Initiatives countering prescription drug abuse range from prevention and treatment to enforcement. These activities include scheduling chemicals used in certain prescription drugs, supporting public awareness campaigns, bolstering law enforcement, and providing assistance to states—in part through PDMPs. This report focuses on PDMPs.

[13] Legislation has been introduced in the 112th Congress that would take up these issues (see, for example, section 1141 of the Food and Drug Administration Safety and Innovation Act (S. 3187), the Medicare and Medicaid FAST Act (H.R. 3399, S. 1251), and ID MEDS Act (H.R. 4292, S. 2254)).

[14] Office of National Drug Control Policy, *Epidemic Responding to America's Prescription Drug Abuse Crisis*, 2011, http://www.whitehouse.gov/sites/default/files/ondcp/issues-content/prescription-drugs/rx_abuse_plan.pdf.

Prescription Drug Monitoring Programs (PDMPs)

PDMPs maintain statewide electronic databases of designated information on specified prescription drugs dispensed within the states. Data are made available to individuals or organizations as authorized under state law; these may include prescribers, law enforcement officials, licensing boards, or others. Possible uses of PDMPs include

- supporting patient access to controlled substances for legitimate medical use;

- identifying or preventing drug abuse and diversion;

- facilitating the identification of prescription drug-addicted individuals and appropriate intervention and treatment;

- outlining use and abuse trends to inform public health initiatives; and

- educating individuals about prescription drug use, abuse, and diversion.[15]

In addition to uses of PDMPs aimed at drug abuse and diversion, an explicit goal of PDMPs is supporting access to controlled substances for legitimate medical use. This may best be understood by viewing PDMPs in comparison to earlier, paper-based programs called multiple-copy prescription programs. For example, in 1914 a New York state law required physicians to use state-issued, serialized, duplicate prescription forms for certain drugs.[16] Similarly, California began a multiple-copy prescription program using triplicate forms for specified narcotics in 1939; it expanded to monitor all schedule II narcotics in 1972 and schedule II non-narcotics in 1981.[17] Studies of multiple-copy prescription programs found that many prescribers did not order the required prescription forms, rendering them unable to prescribe specified controlled substances even when medically appropriate.[18] In addition, the ability to check a patient's prescription history using an electronic PDMP might give prescribers more confidence when considering the use of drugs with high risk of abuse.

As of June 2012, 40 states had operational PDMPs, nine additional states and one territory (Guam) had enacted PDMP legislation (but the programs were not yet operational), and one state (Missouri) had pending PDMP legislation. The District of Columbia has neither an operational PDMP nor PDMP legislation.[19]

---

[15] National Alliance for Model State Drug Laws, *Prescription Drug Monitoring Programs A Brief Overview*, August 17, 2010, http://www.namsdl.org/documents/PMPsBriefOverview8-17-2010.pdf.

[16] Scott M. Fishman et al., "Regulating Opioid Prescribing Through Prescription Monitoring Programs: Balancing Drug Diversion and Treatment of Pain," *Pain Medicine*, vol. 5, no. 3 (2004), pp. 309-324.

[17] Aaron M. Gilson et al , "Time Series Analysis of California's Prescription Monitoring Program: Impact on Prescribing and Multiple Provider Episodes," *Journal of Pain*, vol. 13, no. 2 (2012), pp. 103-111.

[18] Scott M. Fishman et al., "Regulating Opioid Prescribing Through Prescription Monitoring Programs: Balancing Drug Diversion and Treatment of Pain," *Pain Medicine*, vol. 5, no. 3 (2004), pp. 309-324.

[19] Alliance of States with Prescription Monitoring Programs, *Status of Prescription Drug Monitoring Programs (PDMPs)*, June 13, 2012, http://www.pmpalliance.org/pdf/pmpstatustable2012.pdf. For a map, see http://www.pmpalliance.org/pdf/pmpstatusmap2012.pdf.

Program Operation

The entity responsible for administering the PDMP varies by state and may be pharmacy boards, departments of health, professional licensing agencies, law enforcement agencies, substance abuse agencies, or consumer protection agencies. Of the 49 authorized PDMPs, two-thirds are administered by either state pharmacy boards (18) or health departments (15).[20]

Each state determines which entities dispensing prescriptions for controlled substances are required to submit data to the PDMP. These entities can include hospitals and facilities, sole practitioners, or wholesale distributors, among others.[21] Some states also have statutory authority to require out-of-state, mail order, and internet pharmacies to submit data to the PDMP regarding prescription or controlled drugs dispensed to residents of the state. For instance, if a patient in Alabama receives a prescription for a monitored drug from an out-of-state mail order pharmacy, the mail order pharmacy must report the prescription to the Alabama PDMP.[22] State laws also indicate which schedules of controlled substances are monitored under each program (see text box for a brief explanation of schedules), which information about the substances is submitted, the means by which dispensers or dispensaries submit the required information, and the timeframe under which information is submitted.

Access to information contained in the PDMP database is determined by state law and varies by state. The majority of states allow pharmacists and practitioners to access information related to their patients, and some also allow other entities—law enforcement, licensing and regulatory boards, state Medicaid Programs, state medical examiners, and research organization—to access the information under certain circumstances.[24] State laws outline the procedures by which information from the PDMP may be accessed.

> **Schedules of Controlled Substances**
>
> The Controlled Substances Act (21 U.S.C. §801 et seq.) estab ishes schedules for controlled substances (including drugs), ranging from schedule I (most restrictive) to schedule V (least restrictive). Drugs on schedule I have no currently accepted medical use in the United States and are not available by prescription. Drugs with recognized medical uses are on schedules II through V, with each successive schedule representing a lower risk of abuse.[23]

With respect to how the states identify and investigate cases of potential prescription drug diversion or abuse, PDMPs may be classified as *reactive* or *proactive*. In essence, "[s]tates with [r]eactive PDMPs ... generate solicited reports only in response to a specific inquiry made by a prescriber, dispenser, or other party with appropriate authority" while "[s]tates with [p]roactive

---

[20] Alliance of States with Prescription Monitoring Programs, *Prescription Monitoring Frequently Asked Questions (FAQ)*, 2012, http://www.pmpalliance.org/content/prescription-monitoring-frequently-asked-questions-faq.

[21] Alliance of States with Prescription Monitoring Programs, *Prescription Monitoring Program Model Act 2010 Revision*, http://www.pmpalliance.org/pdf/PMPModelActFinal20100628.pdf.

[22] National Alliance for Model State Drug Laws, *States With Statutory Authority to Require Nonresident Pharmacies to Report to Prescription Monitoring Program*, December 28, 2011, http://www.namsdl.org/documents/ ReqmtofMailOrderandNonresidentPharmaciestoReporttoPMP_001.pdf.

[23] For more information, please see CRS Report R40548, *Legal Issues Relating to the Disposal of Dispensed Controlled Substances*, by Brian T. Yeh.

[24] Alliance of States with Prescription Monitoring Programs, *Prescription Monitoring Frequently Asked Questions (FAQ)*, 2012, http://www.pmpalliance.org/content/prescription-monitoring-frequently-asked-questions-faq.

PDMPs ... identify and investigate cases, generating unsolicited reports whenever suspicious behavior is detected."[25]

Interstate Information Sharing and Interoperability

State PDMPs vary widely with respect to whether or how information contained in the database is shared with other states. While some states do not have measures in place allowing interstate sharing of information, others have specific practices for sharing. These practices may be based on factors such as agreed-upon reciprocity between states, or whether a request stems from an ongoing investigation.[26] As of February 2012, 28 states allowed for sharing PDMP information on some level—with PDMPs in other states, with authorized PDMP users in other states, or both.[27]

Researchers have provided states with guidance in creating Memoranda of Understanding (MOUs) for interstate data exchange. Questions that states may consider when drafting an MOU include the following:[28]

- How is the information to be reported?
- How will the information be used by the relevant states?
- What are the guidelines on data retention?
- What are the state responsibilities in the event of a data breach?
- Are there measures in place for conflict resolution?
- What are the consequences of potential data misuse?

In addition, the Council of State Governments has highlighted four areas as central to the success of interstate compacts regarding PDMPs and data sharing:

Education—responsibility of providers, data integrity, training requirements (start up versus ongoing)[;]

Funding—state funding, costs of data sharing, costs of operation[;]

Security and Access—authorized users, authentication, audit trails, Internet access, vendor security, reporting, privacy, confidentiality, use of data[; and]

Technology—data transfer and exchange, uniformity and standards, cost reduction, compatibility, quality/error correction[.][29]

---

[25] Ronald Simeone and Lynn Holland, *Executive Summary An Evaluation of Prescription Drug Monitoring Programs*, Simeone Associates, Inc., http://www.namsdl.org/resources/PDMP%20Study%20Executive%20Summary.pdf.

[26] National Alliance for Model State Drug Laws, *Interstate Sharing of Prescription Monitoring Database Information*, February 8, 2012, http://www.namsdl.org/documents/InterstateSharingofPMPInformation02082012.pdf.

[27] For a map depicting the interstate sharing of PDMP data, see http://www.namsdl.org/documents/ InterstateSharingofPMPData03142012.pdf.

[28] Alliance of States With Prescription Monitoring Programs and Brandeis University's Training and Technical Assistance Center, *Memorandum Of Understanding Writing Guide for States with Prescription Monitoring Programs*, funded through a grant (No. 2010-DG-BX-K088) from the Bureau of Justice Assistance.

[29] The Council of State Governments, National Center for Interstate Compacts, *Prescription Drug Monitoring Programs Interstate Compact—National Advisory Panel*, November 5-6, 2009, http://www.csg.org/pubs/capitolideas/ (continued...)

An effort is ongoing to facilitate information sharing using prescription monitoring information exchange (PMIX) architecture.[30] The PMIX program is intended to enable the interstate exchange of PDMP information, providing information on an individual's prescription drug history across states participating in the information exchange. This information can help identify potential prescription drug abuse or diversion, and can help inform stakeholders such as law enforcement, health and human services, health practitioners, and public regulatory agencies. A state can participate in the PMIX program if it has

- legislation allowing it to share information with other states in real time,

- identified at least one other state as a partner in the information exchange, and

- either (1) established an MOU with their identified partner(s) in the information exchange or (2) ratified the Prescription Monitoring Interstate Compact.[31]

The infrastructure of the PMIX program is based on the National Information Exchange Model, which is a data sharing partnership between all levels of government as well as the private sector.[32] To facilitate information security and data privacy, data are encrypted while passing through "hubs," and no data are actually stored on these hubs. PMIX allows for hubs to exist at the state and national levels, and it allows for hub-to-hub information exchange.[33]

With pharmaceutical industry support, the National Association of Boards of Pharmacy (NABP) has developed a technology platform to facilitate interstate sharing of PDMP data, called InterConnect, which NABP has committed to make compliant with PMIX architecture.[34] NABP anticipates that approximately 20 states will be sharing data using NABP InterConnect by the end of 2012, including 14 that had executed MOUs to participate as of March 2012.[35]

Currently, there are no national level standards for state PDMP information sharing and interoperability. Legislation has been introduced in the 112th Congress that would take up these issues.[36] Some bills would, among other things, examine the current interoperability of state level

---

(...continued)

enews/enewsissue38/21stCenturyHandout.pdf.

[30] More information on PMIX can be found at http://www.pmpalliance.org/content/prescription-monitoring-information-exchange-pmix. A pilot project between Kentucky and Ohio's PDMPs formed the springboard for the larger PMIX initiative. Through this pilot, a PMIX hub server was installed in Ohio, and Ohio and Kentucky signed an MOU for data exchange, http://www.ijis.org/_programs/pdmp.html.

[31] Alliance of States With Prescription Monitoring Programs, *Prescription Monitoring Information Exchange (PMIX)*, http://www.pmpalliance.org/content/prescription-monitoring-information-exchange-pmix. Draft language of the compact is available at http://www.pmpalliance.org/pdf/PMPCompactLanguageDraft2010.pdf.

[32] More information can be found at https://www.niem.gov/.

[33] Alliance of States With Prescription Monitoring Programs, *Prescription Monitoring Program Information Exchange (PMIX) Architecture*, Version 1.0, April 2012, http://www.pmpalliance.org/pdf/PMIX%20National%20Architecture%20Document.pdf.

[34] U.S. Department of Justice, Office of Justice Programs, Bureau of Justice Assistance, BJA Policy on Use of Harold Rogers Prescription Drug Monitoring Program (HRPDMP) Funding to Support Interstate Data Sharing Activities, May 30, 2012, https://www.bja.gov/Programs/PDMPPolicy.pdf. This supersedes interim policy guidance documentation dated March 21, 2012, and April 17, 2012.

[35] National Association of State Boards of Pharmacy (NABP), *Fact Sheet NABP PMP InterConnect*, 2012, http://www.nabp.net/programs/assets/PMPInterconnectFactSheet.pdf.

[36] For example, section 1141 of the Food and Drug Administration Safety and Innovation Act (S. 3187, as passed both House and Senate) would authorize the Secretary of HHS, consulting with the Attorney General as appropriate, to facilitate the development of recommendations on interoperability standards for interstate exchange of PDMP (continued...)

PDMPs,[37] and others would establish national-level standards for the interoperability of state PDMPs receiving federal funding.[38]

Compliance and Enforcement Mechanisms

In ensuring that a given state's PDMP reflects comprehensive data from all relevant pharmacies, physicians, and other dispensaries, one principal concern is how to ensure that these dispensaries are reporting prescription data to the program. The laws or rules governing consequences for failure to report data are determined by each state. For example, one consequence may be disciplinary action by the appropriate licensing board or commission. Another may be that failure to report information could trigger the PDMP program office to report the lapse in compliance to the PDMP governing agency, which may then refer the information to law enforcement.[39]

Program Costs

PDMP expenses involve startup costs, funds needed to operate and maintain the programs, and any monies used to enhance program operation and interoperability. Overall program costs can entail

- hardware such as servers;

- software to run the PDMP database and ensure information security;

- connectivity such that pharmacies and dispensaries can enter data and such that prescribers and/or law enforcement officials can request and access data;

- staff to administer the PDMP and provide technical assistance; and

- overhead fees.

A 2009 evaluation by the Maryland Advisory Council on Prescription Drug Monitoring assessed existing state PDMPs on a range of factors including the costs associated with establishing and maintaining the programs.[40] The overarching finding was that costs vary widely, with program startup costs ranging from $450,000 to over $1.5 million. Further, based on available data from six operational PDMPs, results from the Maryland Advisory Council's evaluation indicate that annual operating costs range from $125,000 to nearly $1.0 million, with an average annual cost of about $500,000. For example, the state of Florida estimated that it would "cost $480,000 dollars

---

(...continued)

information by states receiving federal grants to support their PDMPs.

[37] See, for example, the Medicare and Medicaid FAST Act (H.R. 3399, S. 1251).

[38] See, for example, the ID MEDS Act (H.R. 4292, S. 2254).

[39] See, for example, Florida's PDMP rule states that "Failure to report the dispensing of Schedules II-IV controlled substances will result in the Program filing a complaint with the Department [of Health] for investigation and a referral to law enforcement," Rule 64K-1.004, https://www.flrules.org/gateway/RuleNo.asp?title= Prescription%20Drug%20Monitoring%20Program&ID=64K-1.004.

[40] Maryland Advisory Council on Prescription Drug Monitoring, *Maryland Advisory Council on Prescription Drug Monitoring Legislative Report*, December 31, 2009, p. 76, http://dhmh.maryland.gov/laboratories/drugcont/docs/ Final%20Report%20of%20recommendations%20by%20the%20PDM%20Advisory%20Council%2012-31-09.pdf.

to purchase and initially operate the system for one year" and that "[a]nnual operating costs after that [would be] $450,000 per year."[41]

The Maryland Advisory Council reported that

> [c]ost variations are affected by the frequency of data collection (e.g., daily, weekly, bi-weekly, monthly), the use of third party vendors for data collection and analysis, the number of prescriptions written and filled in the state, the number of drug schedules (II-V) and drugs of interest collected, and the use of official forms or other required collection and submission mechanisms.[42]

A 2002 Government Accountability Office (GAO) evaluation of PDMP costs in Kentucky, Nevada, and Utah revealed findings similar to those presented by the Maryland Advisory Council. GAO noted a number of PDMP design and operational factors driving variations in state costs for running PDMPs. Specifically, these involved "differences in the PDMP systems implemented, the number of pharmacies reporting drug dispensing data, and the number of practitioners and law enforcement agencies seeking information from the systems."[43]

PDMP Financing

States finance the startup and operation of PDMPs through a variety of channels. PDMP financing often involves monies from the state general fund, prescriber and pharmacy licensing fees, state controlled substance registration fees, health insurers' fees, direct-support organizations, state or federal grants, or a combination thereof.[44] Guidelines for how states may fund PDMPs are outlined in each state's PDMP authorizing legislation. For example, Oregon's PDMP has a fund within the state treasury. This fund receives monies, in part, from a proportion of medical provider fees. These fees are paid to the appropriate medical board, and the board in turn transmits a portion of these fees to the PDMP fund. The Oregon Department of Human Services, which administers the PDMP, may also accept and deposit into the fund money from a variety of additional sources, including grants and donations.[45]

Some states prohibit the use of certain sources of funding, thus limiting the potential range of funding mechanisms. For instance, Florida law specifically prohibits the use of state funds or funds received—directly or indirectly—from prescription drug manufacturers to support the

---

[41] Executive Office of the Governor, Florida Office of Drug Control, *Prescription Drug Monitoring Program Frequently Asked Questions*, http://drugcontrol.flgov.com/pdmp/faq.html.

[42] Maryland Advisory Council on Prescription Drug Monitoring, *Maryland Advisory Council on Prescription Drug Monitoring Legislative Report*, December 31, 2009, pp. 76-77. An earlier (2002) evaluation of PDMPs by the Government Accountability Office (GAO) found similar reasons for variability in state costs for PDMP operation. These variations were driven by "differences in the PDMP systems implemented, the number of pharmacies reporting drug dispensing data, and the number of practitioners and law enforcement agencies seeking information from the systems."

[43] U.S. General Accounting Office, *Prescription Drugs State Monitoring Programs Provide Useful Tool to Reduce Diversion*, GAO-02-634, May 2002, p. 3, http://www.gao.gov/assets/240/234687.pdf.

[44] Alliance of States With Prescription Monitoring Programs, *Prescription Monitoring Programs Funding Mechanisms & Business Models*, National Legislation & Implementation Meeting 2010, 2010, p. 3, http://www.pmpalliance.org/pdf/PPTs/LI2010/PMP-FundingBusModels.pdf.

[45] Oregon PDMP statute (ORS 431.960 et seq.), available at http://www.orpdmp.com/orpdmpfiles/PDF_Files/ORS%20431.960%20PDMP.pdf.

PDMP. As such, the program receives funding from three sources: the Florida PDMP Foundation, Inc., an organization established in Florida law for the purpose of funding the PDMP; federal grants; and private grants and donations.[46]

PDMP Effectiveness

The available evidence suggests that PDMPs are effective in some ways for both law enforcement and health care purposes; however, research on the effectiveness of PDMPs is limited, especially in the area of law enforcement. Assessments of effectiveness may also take into consideration potential unintended consequences of PDMPs. Experts suggest that PDMPs have the potential to be more effective.

Effectiveness Research

Research on PDMP effectiveness suggests that existence of a PDMP has an impact on both law enforcement and health care. A 2002 GAO study found that "the time and effort required by law enforcement and regulatory investigators to explore leads and the merits of possible drug diversion cases" declined after PDMP implementation.[47] The study found that Kentucky investigations of alleged doctor shoppers took an average of 156 days prior to PDMP implementation and 16 days after PDMP implementation (a 90% decrease). Nevada and Utah reported decreases in investigation time of 83% and 80%, respectively. These decreases in investigation time do not necessarily translate into less prescription drug abuse.

A 2012 review article summarized all peer-reviewed research articles about PDMPs published between 2001 and 2011, which amounted to 11 articles (not all of which addressed effectiveness).[48] The author concluded that PDMPs reduce "doctor shopping," change prescribing behavior, and reduce prescription drug abuse. For example, a 2006 federally funded study (included in the 2012 review article) found that PDMPs—especially ones that issue reports proactively—change prescriber behavior in a way that reduces the per capita supply of prescription pain relievers and stimulants, which in turn reduces the likelihood of abuse.[49] A study published in 2012 (and therefore not included in the review) found that while opioid abuse was increasing over time, the rate of increase was slower in states with PDMPs than in states without PDMPs.[50]

---

[46] Florida Department of Health, *Funding the E-FORSCE System*, http://www.doh.state.fl.us/mqa/PDMP/funding.html.

[47] U.S. General Accounting Office, *Prescription Drugs State Monitoring Programs Provide Useful Tool to Reduce Diversion*, GAO-02-634, May 2002, p. 3, http://www.gao.gov/assets/240/234687.pdf.

[48] Julie Worley, "Prescription Drug Monitoring Programs, a Response to Doctor Shopping: Purpose, Effectiveness, and Directions for Future Research," *Issues in Mental Health Nursing*, vol. 33, no. 5 (2012), pp. 319-328. Note: The GAO study was not included, because it was not published in the peer-reviewed literature.

[49] Ronald Simeone and Lynn Holland, *An Evaluation of Prescription Drug Monitoring Programs*, Simeone Associates, Inc., No. 2005PMBXK189, September 1, 2006, http://www.simeoneassociates.com/simeone3.pdf. This study was commissioned by the U.S. Department of Justice (DOJ), Office of Justice Programs (OJP), Bureau of Justice Assistance (BJA).

[50] Liza M. Reifler et al., "Do Prescription Monitoring Programs Impact State Trends in Opioid Abuse/Misuse," *Pain Medicine*, no. 13 (2012), pp. 434-442.

Limitations of the Research

Research regarding PDMP effectiveness is limited, at least in part, by the difficulties inherent in conducting such research. Challenges in conducting high-quality research on PDMP effectiveness include (but are not limited to) (1) defining effectiveness, (2) accounting for differences among PDMPs, and (3) considering potential confounding factors.

In order to study effectiveness, researchers must first define effectiveness in a way that can be systematically measured as a study outcome. PDMPs are statewide programs; thus, researchers look for outcome measures that are available statewide. Some outcomes that have been measured in research on PDMP effectiveness are shipment and sales of controlled substances, benzodiazepine use in a Medicaid population, opioid consumption, substance abuse treatment admissions, drug overdose mortality, and multiple provider episodes (i.e., doctor shopping).[51] On the one hand, opioid consumption includes both nonmedical use of opioids and medically appropriate use of opioids to manage pain. On the other hand, a count of substance abuse treatment admissions fails to capture substance abuse that goes untreated. Each of these measures presents only a portion of the picture of prescription drug diversion and abuse.

Studies that compare states with and without PDMPs and/or before and after implementation of a PDMP vary in the degree to which they account for differences among PDMPs. For example, despite evidence that proactive PDMPs are more effective than reactive PDMPs, most studies do not distinguish between proactive and reactive PDMPs. Another difference that may influence PDMP effectiveness is in which drugs are required to be reported to the PDMP, ranging from only those drugs with the highest potential for abuse to all prescription controlled substances plus other drugs of concern. Research generally focuses on those controlled substances that are included in all of the PDMPs being examined. Differences in PDMPs over time may also influence effectiveness. For example, some states have transitioned from paper-based systems for monitoring prescriptions for controlled substances to the electronic PDMPs used today. Effectiveness studies have generally not accounted for such transitions over time, classifying two different systems as the same PDMP. Accounting for these and other differences between PDMPs may shed light on factors that influence effectiveness.

Researchers must also consider factors that may confound study results, both when comparing outcomes across states (i.e., those with and without PDMPs) and when comparing outcomes over time (i.e., before and after PDMP implementation). For example, the baseline rate of prescription drug abuse may vary across states; the authors of the federally funded study noted that the likelihood of abuse was actually higher in states with PDMPs than in states without PDMPs, but that proactive PDMPs inhibited the rate of increase in prescription drug abuse.[52] A PDMP may be part of a larger effort to reduce prescription drug diversion and abuse, in which case other initiatives may be responsible for any change in the outcome. A seemingly unrelated event, such as an economic downturn or upturn, may also affect the outcome. These considerations, among

---

[51] See summaries of several studies conducted between 2001 and 2011 in Julie Worley, "Prescription Drug Monitoring Programs, a Response to Doctor Shopping: Purpose, Effectiveness, and Directions for Future Research," *Issues in Mental Health Nursing*, vol. 33, no. 5 (2012), pp. 319-328; see also Liza M. Reifler et al., "Do Prescription Monitoring Programs Impact State Trends in Opioid Abuse/Misuse," *Pain Medicine*, vol. 13, no. 3 (2012), pp. 434-442; and Aaron M. Gilson et al., "Time Series Analysis of California's Prescription Monitoring Program: Impact on Prescribing and Multiple Provider Episodes," *Journal of Pain*, vol. 13, no. 2 (2012), pp. 103-111.

[52] Ronald Simeone and Lynn Holland, *An Evaluation of Prescription Drug Monitoring Programs*, Simeone Associates, Inc., No. 2005PMBXK189, September 1, 2006, http://www.simeoneassociates.com/simeone3.pdf.

many others, impede the ability of researchers—and therefore policymakers—to draw conclusions about the effectiveness of PDMPs.

Potential Unintended Consequences

PDMPs may have unintended consequences beyond reducing prescription drug diversion and abuse.[53] Prescribers may hesitate to prescribe medications monitored by the PDMP—even for appropriate medical use—if they are concerned about potentially coming under scrutiny from law enforcement or licensing authorities. Studies of paper-based prescription monitoring programs that preceded the electronic PDMPs found that many prescribers did not order the required prescription forms, rendering them unable to prescribe specified controlled substances at all. Their concerns may lead prescribers to replace medications that are monitored by the PDMP with medications that are not monitored by the PDMP, even if the unmonitored medications are inferior in terms of effectiveness or side effects. Studies showed that after benzodiazepines were added to New York's paper-based program in 1989, a decrease in benzodiazepine prescriptions was accompanied by an increase in prescriptions for other sedatives. Individuals whose intent is to use controlled substances for nonmedical purposes may also substitute unmonitored prescription drugs or street drugs for those that are monitored by the PDMP.

Like prescribers, patients may fear coming under scrutiny from law enforcement if they use medications monitored by the PDMP, even if they have a legitimate medical need for the medications. Patients may worry about changes in prescribing behavior, which may limit their access to needed medications. Patients may worry about the additional cost of more frequent office visits if prescribers become more cautious about writing prescriptions with refills. Patients may also have concerns about the privacy and security of their prescription information if it is submitted to a PDMP.

Another potential unintended consequence of a state PDMP is that it may push drug diversion activities over the border into a neighboring state with no PDMP. A GAO study, completed in 2002, found evidence of this spillover across state lines.[54] This concern is one of the reasons interstate data sharing and interoperability have become priorities. Similarly, a PDMP may push drug diversion activities into a neighboring state with a PDMP that does not monitor as many medications. In any of these cases, the effectiveness of the PDMP may be offset by unintended consequences.

A PDMP may also have positive unintended consequences. For example, when accessing information from a PDMP, a prescriber or dispenser may identify a patient who is receiving legitimate prescriptions for multiple controlled substances and who is therefore at risk of harmful drug interactions.[55] PDMPs may also enable prescribers to monitor their own DEA number to determine whether someone else is using it to forge prescriptions.[56]

---

[53] Most of the unintended consequences identified in this section are discussed in Scott M. Fishman et al., "Regulating Opioid Prescribing Through Prescription Monitoring Programs: Balancing Drug Diversion and Treatment of Pain," *Pain Medicine*, vol. 5, no. 3 (2004), pp. 309-324.

[54] U.S. General Accounting Office, *Prescription Drugs State Monitoring Programs Provide Useful Tool to Reduce Diversion*, GAO-02-634, May 2002, p. 3, http://www.gao.gov/assets/240/234687.pdf.

[55] Jeanmarie Perrone and Lewis S. Nelson, "Medication Reconciliation for Controlled Substances—An "Ideal" Prescription-Drug Monitoring Program," *New England Journal of Medicine*, vol. 366, no. 25 (2012), p. 2341-2343.

[56] Ibid.

Potential to Increase Effectiveness

A PDMP is essentially a source of information; its effectiveness depends largely on the quality of the information and how the information is used.[57] The quality of PDMP information depends on its timeliness, completeness, accuracy, and consistency. Expert recommendations to enhance data quality include

- collecting data at the point of sale (in real time);

- monitoring all prescribed controlled substances and other drugs of concern;

- integrating electronic prescribing technology;

- sharing data between states;

- standardizing the content across states;

- identifying the person picking up the prescription (which may be someone other than the patient, such as a family member); and

- linking prescription records for an individual (to avoid confusion if, for example, an address changes or a name is spelled differently).

In order for PDMP information to be well used, it must be accessible. A survey of prescribers found that the most common reason given for not using a PDMP was the time required to access it (73%); two other reasons—difficult navigation of the web portal (29%) and forgetting the password (28%)—may contribute to the amount of time required to access PDMP information. More than a third of survey respondents (39%) felt that accessing PDMP information would not change their practice for that patient, although research suggests PDMP information changes prescribing behavior. Relatively small numbers of respondents reported that lack of computer availability (9%) or never having applied for access (11%) were barriers to using a PDMP.[58] Expert recommendations to enhance data use include

- providing easy online access;

- issuing automated, unsolicited reports; and

- increasing participation through education and promotional campaigns.

Experts recommend making PDMP information available for research and public health purposes, which would require permitting access by designated non-prescribers (e.g., researchers and medical examiners). An example of a public health use of PDMP information is to identify patients for enrollment in special programs: Washington state used its PDMP to select Medicaid enrollees for a Patient Review Coordination Program, which decreased emergency department visits, physician visits, and prescriptions (resulting in an average savings of $6,000 per patient per

---

[57] Unless otherwise indicated, recommendations in this section are drawn from two sources: (1) Prescription Monitoring Program Center of Excellence at Brandeis University, "A New Generation of Prescription Monitoring Programs: Adopting Best Practices," presentation at Harold Rogers PDMP National Meeting, Washington, DC, June 4-6, 2012; and (2) Jeanmarie Perrone and Lewis S. Nelson, "Medication Reconciliation for Controlled Substances—An "Ideal" Prescription-Drug Monitoring Program," *New England Journal of Medicine*, vol. 366, no. 25 (2012), p. 2341-2343.

[58] Jeanmarie Perrone and Lewis S. Nelson, "Medication Reconciliation for Controlled Substances—An "Ideal" Prescription-Drug Monitoring Program," *New England Journal of Medicine*, vol. 366, no. 25 (2012), p. 2341-2343.

---

year).[59] PDMP data may also be analyzed to identify geographic areas where interventions (such as increased law enforcement attention or establishment of a substance abuse clinic) are most needed. Carefully controlled access to de-identified data for research and public health purposes may yield other uses.

Federal Grant Programs for State PDMPs

The federal government has established two grant programs aimed at supporting state PDMPs—the Harold Rogers PDMP and the National All Schedules Prescription Electronic Reporting Act of 2005 (P.L. 109-60, NASPER). The sections that follow provide an overview of each program.

Harold Rogers PDMP

The Harold Rogers PDMP is a discretionary, competitive grant program administered by the U.S. Department of Justice (DOJ), Office of Justice Programs (OJP), Bureau of Justice Assistance (BJA). It was created to help law enforcement, regulatory entities, and public health officials analyze data on prescriptions for controlled substances.[60] Law enforcement uses of PDMP data include (but are not limited to) investigations of physicians who prescribe controlled substances for drug dealers or abusers, pharmacists who falsify records in order to sell controlled substances, and people who forge prescriptions.[61]

The program assists states (including U.S. territories) in the planning, implementation, and enhancement of their PDMPs. This involves

- establishing data collection and analysis systems to bolster the drug abuse prevention efforts of law enforcement, regulatory entities, and public health officials;

- enhancing existing PDMPs' use of data in order to identity trends in drug abuse and sources of diversion as well as increase the number of PDMP users;

- participating in national efforts to evaluate the efficiency and effectiveness of PDMPs;

- implementing and enhancing the interstate exchange of information to prevent diversion;

- assessing the efficiency and effectiveness of existing PDMPs and encouraging other states to implement programs; and

- enhancing collaboration between law enforcement, prosecutors, treatment professionals, medical community members, and pharmacies to create a comprehensive PDMP strategy.[62]

---

[59] Washington state update presented at Harold Rogers PDMP National Meeting, Washington, DC, June 4-6, 2012.

[60] More information on this program can be found at from the U.S. Department of Justice, Bureau of Justice Assistance, *Harold Rogers Prescription Drug Monitoring Program*, http://www.ojp.usdoj.gov/BJA/grant/prescripdrugs.html.

[61] U.S. Department of Justice, Drug Enforcement Administration, Office of Diversion Control, http://www.deadiversion.usdoj.gov.

[62] U.S. Department of Justice, Office of Justice Programs, Bureau of Justice Assistance, *Harold Rogers Prescription* (continued...)

Grant Purpose Areas

States may apply for Harold Rogers PDMP grants in one of three categories: planning, implementation, or enhancement.[63]

- **Planning Grants.** States that do not have an operational PDMP may apply for planning grants of up to $50,000, regardless of whether they have regulations or legislation requiring a PDMP.

- **Implementation Grants.** States with legislation or regulations requiring the centralized collection of prescription drug dispensing data and/or designating the oversight or implementation of such a PDMP to a state agency may apply for implementation grants of up to $400,000.

- **Enhancement Grants.** States seeking to enhance or expand their existing PDMPs may apply for enhancement grants of up to $400,000.

PDMP conformance to prescription monitoring information exchange (PMIX) architecture is an explicit goal of BJA, and grant funding may be used for implementation of PMIX architecture-compliant hub solutions (among other things).[64]

Appropriations

The program began receiving federal funding in FY2002 through the Departments of Commerce, Justice, and State, the Judiciary, and Related Agencies Appropriations Act, 2002 (P.L. 107-77). While the program itself has never been authorized in statute, funding for the program has been provided to DOJ each year through the annual appropriations process. Annual appropriations information is listed in **Table 1.**

Table 1. Harold Rogers Prescription Drug Monitoring Program Funding

(In millions of dollars)

Fiscal Year	Appropriation
2002	$2.00
2003	$7.50
2004	$7.00
2005	$10.00
2006	$7.50
2007	$7.50

(...continued)

Drug Monitoring Program FY 2010 Competitive Grant Announcement, p. 1, http://www.ojp.usdoj.gov/BJA/grant/10PDMPsol.pdf.

[63] Ibid., pp. 2 – 3.

[64] U.S. Department of Justice, Office of Justice Programs, Bureau of Justice Assistance, BJA Policy on Use of Harold Rogers Prescription Drug Monitoring Program (HRPDMP) Funding to Support Interstate Data Sharing Activities, May 30, 2012, https://www.bja.gov/Programs/PDMPPolicy.pdf. This supersedes interim policy guidance documentation dated March 21, 2012, and April 17, 2012.

Fiscal Year	Appropriation
2008	$7.05
2009	$7.00
2010	$7.00
2011	$5.80
2012	$7.00

Source: FY2002 data from P.L. 107-77; FY2003 data from P.L. 108-7; FY2004 data from P.L. 108-199; FY2005 data from P.L. 108-447; FY2006 data from P.L. 109-108; FY2007 data from P.L. 110-5; FY2008 data from P.L. 110-161; FY2009 data from P.L. 111-8; FY2010 data from P.L. 111-117; FY2011 data are based on CRS analysis of the text of P.L. 112-10; FY2012 data from P.L. 112-55.

National All Schedules Prescription Electronic Reporting Act of 2005 (NASPER)

The NASPER PDMP grant is a formula grant administered by the Department of Health and Human Services (HHS), Substance Abuse and Mental Health Services Administration (SAMHSA), Center for Substance Abuse Treatment (CSAT). The National All Schedules Prescription Electronic Reporting Act of 2005[65] amended the Public Health Service Act[66] to require the Secretary of HHS to award grants to states[67] to establish or improve PDMPs. Specifically, NASPER is intended to provide grant support to states to establish PDMPs that will allow health care providers to access prescription history information in order to identify patients at risk for addiction. It also requires that local, state, and federal law enforcement agencies have access to the database. Of note, however, the grants to states under NASPER are only for the PDMP; they do not fund any substance abuse treatment services.

Grant Purpose Areas

The two objectives of NASPER are to (1) foster the establishment of state-administered PDMPs that providers can access for the early identification of patients at risk for addiction in order to initiate appropriate interventions, and (2) establish a set of best practices for new PDMPs and improvement of existing PDMPs.

Appropriations

Funding was authorized for NASPER beginning in FY2006. The program began receiving appropriations in FY2009. The final continuing resolution for FY2011 (P.L. 112-10) specifically prohibited the funding of NASPER.[68] Annual authorizations of appropriations and actual appropriations are listed in **Table 2**.

---

[65] Unless otherwise noted, all information in this section on NASPER comes from the text of P.L. 109-60.

[66] 42 U.S.C. §280g et seq.

[67] States are defined as each of the 50 states and the District of Columbia

[68] Department of Defense and Full-Year Continuing Appropriations Act, 2011 (P.L. 112-10 §1815(a)(2)).

In order to be eligible for NASPER grant funding, states must meet certain requirements, such as having legal authority to implement PDMPs. All states that submit applications and meet the requirements receive grants non-competitively. The amount awarded to each state is defined by a two-part formula:

1. Each state receives a base amount of 1% of the total funding (i.e., $20,000 in FY2010).

2. The remaining amount is distributed according to the ratio of the number of pharmacies in the individual state to the number of pharmacies in all states with approved applications.

Thirteen states received grants under NASPER in FY2010, the last year of funding.[69]

Table 2. National All Schedules Prescription Electronic Reporting Act of 2005 (NASPER) Funding through FY2012

(In millions of dollars)

Fiscal Year	Authorization of Appropriation	Appropriation
2006	$15.00	$0.00
2007	$15.00	$0.00
2008	$10.00	$0.00
2009	$10.00	$2.00
2010	$10.00	$2.00
2011	NA	$0.00
2012	NA	$0.00

Source: Authorizations of appropriations through FY2010 from P.L. 109-60. Appropriations through FY2010 from Department of Health and Human Services, Fiscal Year 2011, Substance Abuse and Mental Health Services Administration, Justification of Estimates for Appropriations Committees. Appropriations for FY2011 from P.L. 112-10. Appropriations for FY2012 from P.L. 112-74.

Note: NA = not authorized.

Program Comparison

Table 3 provides an overview and comparison of the Harold Rogers PDMP and the NASPER PDMP. Basic information is provided on program legislation, administering agencies, program objectives, performance measures, grant types, authorization of appropriations, and actual appropriations.

---

[69] U.S. Department of Health and Human Services, *TAGGS - Tracking Accountability in Government Grants System*, http://taggs.hhs.gov/AdvancedSearch.cfm.

Table 3. Comparison of the Harold Rogers Prescription Drug Monitoring Program (PDMP) and the National All Schedules Prescription Electronic Reporting Act of 2005 (NASPER)

	Harold Rogers	NASPER
Legislation	Departments of Commerce, Justice, and State, the Judiciary, and Related Agencies Appropriations Act, 2002 (P.L. 107-77)	National All Schedules Prescription Electronic Reporting Act of 2005 (P.L. 109-60)
Administering Agency	U.S. Department of Justice (DOJ), Office of Justice Programs (OJP), Bureau of Justice Assistance (BJA)	U.S. Department of Health and Human Services (HHS), Substance Abuse and Mental Health Services Administration (SAMHSA), Center for Substance Abuse Treatment (CSAT)
Program Objectives	Help states to plan, implement, and enhance their PDMPs.	Two objectives: 1. Foster the establishment of state-administered PDMPs that providers can access for the early identification of patients at risk for addiction in order to initiate appropriate interventions. 2. Estab ish a set of best practices for new programs and improvement of existing programs.
Grant Funding	Discretionary, competitive grants with three categories: planning, implementation, enhancement.	Formula grant program in which each state with an approved application receives funding according to the following two-part formula: 1. Each state receives a base amount of 1% of the total funding. 2. The remaining amount is distributed according to the ratio of the number of pharmacies in the individual state to the number of pharmacies in all states with approved applications. The HHS Secretary may adjust the amount allocated to a state, after taking into consideration the estimated cost of the state's PDMP.
Authorization of Appropriations	While the program itse f has never been authorized in statute, funding for the program has been provided to DOJ each year since FY2002 through the annual appropriations process.	Authorizes to be appropriated $15.00M per year from FY2006–FY2007 and $10.00M per year from FY2008–FY2010.
Appropriations	Appropriated $2.00M in FY2002, $7.50M in FY2003, $7.00M in FY2004, $10.00M in FY2005, $7.50M in FY2006, $7.50M in FY2007, $7.05M in FY2008, $7.00M in FY2009, $7.00M in FY2010, $5.8M in FY2011, and $7.00M in FY2012.	No funds were appropriated for FY2006–FY2008; appropriated $2.00M per year in FY2009 and FY2010; funding prohibited in final continuing resolution for FY2011. No funds were appropriated for FY2012.

Source: CRS summary of information from the following sources:
For the Harold Rogers PDMP, CRS summary of U.S. Department of Justice, Bureau of Justice Assistance, *Harold Rogers Prescription Drug Monitoring Program*, http://www.ojp.usdoj.gov/BJA/grant/prescripdrugs.html, P.L. 107-77, P.L. 108-7, P.L. 108-199, P.L. 108-447, P.L. 109-108, P.L. 110-5, P.L. 110-161, P.L. 111-8, P.L. 111-117, CRS analysis of the text of P.L. 112-10, and P.L. 112-55.
For NASPER, CRS summary of the National All Schedules Prescription Electronic Reporting Act of 2005 (P.L. 109-60); Department of Health and Human Services, Fiscal Year 2011, Substance Abuse and Mental Health Services Administration, Justification of Estimates for Appropriations Committees; P.L. 112-10 Sec.1815(a)(2); and P.L. 112-74.

Selected Policy Issues

Role of PDMPs in the Federal Prescription Drug Abuse Strategy

In response to the trend in prescription drug abuse, in April 2011 the Obama Administration released an action plan to respond to the "epidemic."[70] This plan, from ONDCP, outlines four primary areas that may reduce the abuse of prescription drugs: educating individuals on the safe use of prescription drugs and risks involved in abusing them; implementing prescription drug monitoring programs (PDMPs) in the states and encouraging information sharing; developing programs for proper drug disposal; and providing law enforcement with tools to enforce proper prescribing practices and disband pill mills.

As part of this plan, the Administration outlined actions to improve the functioning of state PDMPs and increase interstate PDMP operability and communications. Specific actions offered include

- working with states to establish effective PDMPs and encouraging research on PDMP effectiveness and means to improve PDMP effectiveness;

- supporting the NASPER reauthorization;

- ensuring that the Secretaries of the Department of Veterans Affairs (VA)[71] and the Department of Defense (DOD)[72] are authorized to share patient information with state PDMPs;

- encouraging federally funded health care programs to provide controlled substance prescription information to the state PDMPs (in states where they operate health care facilities or pharmacies);

- potentially reimbursing prescribers for checking PDMPs before writing controlled substance prescriptions to patients covered under insurance plans;

- evaluating programs that require certain doctor shoppers or drug abusing individuals to use one doctor and one pharmacy;

- evaluating the potential for state PDMPs to reduce Medicare and Medicaid fraud;

- issuing a final rule from DEA on electronic prescribing of controlled substances;

- increasing the use of "Screening, Brief Intervention, and Referral to Treatment" programs to identify and prevent prescription drug abuse;

---

[70] Office of National Drug Control Policy, *Epidemic Responding to America's Prescription Drug Abuse Crisis*, 2011, http://www.whitehouse.gov/sites/default/files/ondcp/issues-content/prescription-drugs/rx_abuse_plan.pdf.

[71] The Consolidated Appropriations Act, 2012 (P.L. 112-74) authorized the VA Secretary to share prescription information with state PDMPs.

[72] According to Department of Defense, *Report to Congress Medication Management for Physically and Psychologically Wounded Armed Forces Members In Fiscal Year 2011-2012*, RefID: 6-B74CA6F, March 14, 2012, "DoD providers can access PDMPs for controlled substance prescription histories before generating prescriptions for controlled substances.... The military specific response to this challenge includes work by the PharmacoVigilence Center to apply the lessons learned and apply it to the military where relevant." The report does not indicate whether DoD dispensers contribute information to state PDMPs; however, if servicemembers fill prescriptions at retail pharmacies in the private sector (in a state with a PDMP), the prescriptions would be reported just like any others.

- identifying how health information technologies can enhance prescription drug information;

- testing the Centers for Disease Control and Prevention's surveillance system to generate measures of prescription drug abuse;

- assessing the use of the Drug Abuse Warning Network in the domain of prescription drug abuse;

- expanding DOJ's efforts to enhance interstate PDMP interoperability, particularly though the PMIX program; and

- evaluating existing databases with information on prescription drug access, use, misuse, and toxicity.[73]

As noted, supporting PDMPs is just one component in the overall federal efforts against prescription drug abuse. Research on PDMP effectiveness has yielded sometimes inconclusive results, though research findings suggest that PDMPs may contribute to reduced doctor shopping and prescription drug abuse. As such, policymakers may question the extent to which ONDCP, along with the other relevant departments and agencies, has taken steps to accomplish these PDMP-related goals laid out in the Administration's action plan.

Balancing Stakeholder Concerns

While establishment and enhancement of PDMPs (such as interstate data sharing and real-time data access) enjoy broad support,[74] some stakeholders express concerns about (1) health care versus law enforcement uses of PDMP data, particularly with regard to protection of personally identifiable health information, and (2) maintaining access to medication for patients with legitimate medical needs.

Research has demonstrated that PDMPs save law enforcement officials time in investigations, *if law enforcement officials have access to PDMP information*. Concerns about potential law enforcement uses of PDMP data are expressed by stakeholder organizations representing prescribers. The American Medical Association (AMA), a professional association of more than 200,000 physicians, supports the use of PDMPs and recommends that PDMPs be housed in health-related agencies (rather than law enforcement agencies).[75] AMA further recommends that information from PDMPs "be used first for education of the specific physicians involved prior to any civil action against these physicians."[76] The American Society of Addiction Medicine (ASAM), one of several national medical specialty societies under the AMA umbrella, likewise

---

[73] The White House, *Epidemic Responding to America's Prescription Drug Abuse Crisis*, 2011, pp. 6-7, http://www.whitehouse.gov/sites/default/files/ondcp/policy-and-research/rx_abuse_plan.pdf.

[74] For example, the Pharmaceutical Research and Manufacturers of America (PhRMA)—the industry group representing pharmaceutical research and biotechnology companies—supports PDMPs and recommends assessing their effectiveness and exploring enhancements. PhRMA, *Prescription Drug Abuse*, http://www.phrma.org/issues/prescription-drug-abuse.

[75] American Medical Association (AMA), *The AMA Equation Illustrated. 2011 Annual Report*, p. 25, http://www.ama-assn.org/resources/doc/about-ama/2011-annual-report.pdf; AMA Advocacy Resource Center, *Drug Diversion and Prescription Drug Monitoring Programs*, 2012, http://www.ama-assn.org/resources/doc/washington/prescription-drug-monitoring-issue-brief.pdf.

[76] AMA Advocacy Resource Center, *Drug Diversion and Prescription Drug Monitoring Programs*, 2012, http://www.ama-assn.org/resources/doc/washington/prescription-drug-monitoring-issue-brief.pdf.

---

expresses concern about the use of PDMP data for purposes other than health care: "[L]aw enforcement, the judiciary, corrections professionals, employers, and others outside of the health care system should not be granted access to PDMP data except via the means available to them to secure access to other personally identifiable health information."[77] The fact that PDMPs contain personally identifiable health information raises concerns about privacy and data security. Both AMA and ASAM stress the need to subject PDMP information to the same standards applied to other patient records.[78]

Limiting access to medication for patients with legitimate medical need is a potential unintended consequence of PDMP implementation. The prescription drug abuse prevention strategy of the Center for Lawful Access and Abuse Deterrence (CLAAD), which is endorsed by more than 20 organizations, emphasizes that "efforts to prevent abuse must not impede proper medical practice and patient care."[79] The American Academy of Pain Medicine (AAPM), a national medical specialty society under the AMA umbrella, similarly recognizes "the need for policies that support effective control of drug abuse without harming the appropriate treatment of pain."[80] This concern may be related to fears about law enforcement uses of PDMP information, if prescribers are hesitant to prescribe monitored drugs for fear of becoming targets of investigations.

Federal Role in Interstate Information Sharing and Interoperability

In 2012, Administration and congressional attention to PDMPs has largely focused on enhancing interstate information sharing and the interoperability of state systems. The PDMP component of the Administration's action plan to counter prescription drug abuse includes efforts to improve the functioning of state PDMPs and increase interstate PDMP operability and communications. Some bills in the 112th Congress would build on the current system of state PDMPs by establishing standards for information exchange among states.[81] Others would direct certain agencies to examine the current interoperability among state PDMPs.[82]

---

[77] American Society of Addiction Medicine (ASAM), *Public Policy Statement on Measures to Counteract Prescription Drug Diversion, Misuse and Addiction*, January 25, 2012, http://www.asam.org/advocacy/find-a-policy-statement/view-policy-statement/public-policy-statements/2012/01/26/measures-to-counteract-prescription-drug-diversion-misuse-and-addiction.

[78] AMA Advocacy Resource Center, *Drug Diversion and Prescription Drug Monitoring Programs*, 2012, http://www.ama-assn.org/resources/doc/washington/prescription-drug-monitoring-issue-brief.pdf; and ASAM, *Public Policy Statement on Measures to Counteract Prescription Drug Diversion, Misuse and Addiction*, January 25, 2012, http://www.asam.org/advocacy/find-a-policy-statement/view-policy-statement/public-policy-statements/2012/01/26/measures-to-counteract-prescription-drug-diversion-misuse-and-addiction.

[79] Center for Lawful Access and Abuse Deterrence (CLAAD), *National Prescription Drug Abuse Prevention Strategy 2011-2012 Update*, http://www.claad.org/downloads/CLAAD_Strategy2011_v3.pdf. CLAAD is a 501(c)(3) not-for-profit organization that attempts to foster collaboration among health professionals, law enforcement, businesses, government, and other organizations involved in the issue of prescription drug abuse. See CLAAD, *Overview*, http://www.claad.org/about-claad/overview.

[80] American Academy of Pain Medicine (AAPM), *Advocacy Affecting Health Care on Behalf of our Pain Patients*, http://www.painmed.org/advocacy/main.aspx.

[81] See, for example, the Interstate Drug Monitoring Efficiency and Data Sharing (ID MEDS) Act (H.R. 4292, S. 2254).

[82] For example, section 1141 of the Food and Drug Administration Safety and Innovation Act (S. 3187, as passed both House and Senate) would authorize the Secretary of HHS, consulting with the Attorney General as appropriate, to facilitate the development of recommendations on interoperability standards for interstate exchange of PDMP information by states receiving federal grants to support their PDMPs. See also, for example, the Medicare and Medicaid FAST Act (H.R. 3399, S. 1251).

While the majority of proposals in the 112th Congress would focus on enhancing state-level databases and interstate information sharing, others have suggested establishing a national system. For instance, some proposals would establish a national web portal through which practitioners who prescribe or dispense controlled substances would be required to enter information.[83] Some may argue that monitoring controlled prescription substances is a state level activity, along with regulation of pharmacies and licensing of health care professionals. Others may note that with the increasing reliance on mail order prescriptions and online pharmacies that deliver across state lines, monitoring of controlled prescription substances may be evolving into more of a federal or shared state-federal activity. Policymakers may debate the role of the federal government in incentivizing, directing, or establishing PDMP interoperability and information sharing standards and programs. Such a debate could take place in the context of other federal, state, and local efforts to reduce prescription drug abuse.

Author Contact Information

Kristin M. Finklea
Specialist in Domestic Security
kfinklea@crs.loc.gov, 7-6259

Erin Bagalman
Analyst in Health Policy
ebagalman@crs.loc.gov, 7-5345

Lisa N. Sacco
Analyst in Illicit Drugs and Crime Policy
lsacco@crs.loc.gov, 7-7359

---

[83] See, for example, the Fraudulent Prescription Prevention Act of 2011 (H.R. 1266). The database that would be established by this bill might be considered a federal PDMP, although that term is not used in the legislation.